Paleo Diet Cookbook

The Essentials Guide To Paleo Diet That Helps You To Lose Weight, Build Muscle And Live Healthier

Brian Burton

TERMS & CONDITIONS

No part of this book should be transmitted or reproduced in any form whatsoever, including electronic, print, scanning, photocopying, recording or mechanical without the prior written permission of the author. All the information, ideas and guidelines are for educational purpose only. The writer has tried to ensure the utmost accuracy of the content provided in the book, all the readers are advised to follow instructions at their own risk. The author of this book cannot be held liable for any incidental damage, personal or even commercial caused by misrepresentation of the information given in the book. Readers are encouraged to seek professional help when needed.

Table of Contents

Chapter 1: The advantages of The Paleo Diet & The Criticism of The Diet

I am assuming you probably know something about paleo diet. We'll be jumping to specifics.

The advantages of the Paleo diet

The Paleo diet provides you so many health advantages, including:

- **Includes healthy fats:** The Paleo diet includes healthy fats from sources such as seafood, ghee, coconuts, butter, grass-fed meat & poultry. Healthy fats are needed reducing systemic inflammation & maintaining healthy skin, healthy arteries & brain function.
- **The diet is rich in nutrients:** The Paleo diet eliminates processed supplements & carbs it with healthy fats, seeds, nuts, berries, fruits & vegetables. All of these are full of minerals & vitamins.
- **Sustained weight loss:** Most dieters experience muscle growth & body fat loss when doing exercise regularly & following the Paleo diet.

- **The diet includes unprocessed, real food:** The Paleo diet includes unprocessed, real foods. With the diet, you eliminate a whole range of additives, preservatives, coloring, artificial flavoring, sodium & hidden sugars. Not only you lose weight, but also you become healthier.
- **You feel less hungry:** Rich foods & unlike carb, meals that include protein & fat are very satiating. The slow releasing energy from low GI carbs protein & fat help your body to stay active all day without feeling excessively hungry.
- **Reduced bloat:** The diet provides your body enough fiber, which improves digestion & also, the diet improves the gut flora & keeps it healthy.

Criticisms of the Paleo diet

Despite the advantages, there are a few criticisms of the Paleo diet, including

- **You've to follow strictly to get the result:** To get the main advantages of the diet, you've to follow it strictly; otherwise, the diet would not work.

- **The diet is expensive:** The Paleo diet includes unprocessed, natural, nutrient dense foods, which are expensive.

- **The diet is harder to follow:** To strictly follow the Paleo diet, you've to cook. However, we're living a busy life these days & have no time to cook & this makes the diet hard to follow.

- **There is no standard Paleo diet:** When eating Paleo, we follow the diet of our hunter-gatherer ancestors. However, our ancestors lived in different parts of the world, including coastal areas, islands, desert areas or maybe arctic condition. **Different part of the world offers different types of foods & this is why there is no standard Paleo diet**.

Chapter 2: What to Eat on Paleo Diet

The list of products you may eat on paleo diet is very extensive. Here it's:

- Despite the fact that in the Paleo Age gelatin was not present, the paleo adepts use it for cooking. In the latest versions of the diet, butter is also allowed.
- Sea salt, spices & natural seasonings.
- Fish & seafood caught in the rivers, seas, oceans.
- Eggs of quails, chickens, ostriches, grown naturally.
- Fruits: apricots, avocados, bananas, lime , kiwi, tangerines , lemons, pears , grapes, oranges, pineapple, mango , figs, melon, watermelon, passion fruit & papaya, etc. grown without the use of fertilizers.
- Water, infusions of herbs, coconut milk are allowed for drinks. Some include alcohol & coffee in small amounts.
- Berries: raspberries, blackberries, blueberries, strawberries, cranberries, cherries, etc. grown without the use of fertilizers.
- Soy sauce & apple cider vinegar (naturally fermented without addition of wheat)

- Allowed fats: avocado oil, linseed oil, macadamia nut oil, olive oil, walnut oil & coconut oil (only in small amounts).
- Vegetables: cauliflower, cabbage, zucchini, asparagus, broccoli, spinach, artichokes, carrots, green onions, celery, etc. grown without the use of fertilizers.
- Nuts: pecans, almonds, cashews, pine, hazelnuts, nuts, walnuts, sunflower seeds & pumpkin seeds, except for peanuts, as they are a representative of legumes.
- Mushrooms.
- Meat: lamb, rabbit, pork, venison, poultry, bacon, veal, beef. The strictest followers use only meat of wild birds, animals or maybe organic meat obtained by growing animals without the use of supplements, etc.

Chapter 3: What Not to Eat on Paleo Diet

The following products are not allowed in the paleo diet:

- All products with soybean content.
- Legumes: lentils, beans , peas, peanuts, soybeans contain phytates & lectin, which slow down digestion or maybe even completely remove such useful elements from the body as magnesium, iron , zinc & calcium.
- Alcohol, coffee, tea , drinks, packaged juices.
- Yeast, salt, vinegar.
- Artificial fats, convenience foods, fast food, spread, margarine & products in packages labeled "fat-free"and"dietary".
- In the original version of Paleo diet there is no place for dairy products & milk. The human body is ill adapted to absorb milk, which is why casein & lactose intolerance is so often experienced. Nuts, cabbage & coconut milk may be considered as a source of calcium.
- Artificial sweeteners, sugar & the whole group of products with their content.
- All cereals without exception: flour, pasta, cereals, grains & bread. According to me, cereals at main don't do any good, at worst -

they may only do much harm. Most grains contain gluten, which contributes to the destruction of the intestinal flora, provokes the emergence of bacterial infections, inhibits the absorption of vitamins. A certain group of lectins, contained in legumes & cereals, reduces weakens the immune system & intestinal absorbency.

- The list of prohibited products also includes potatoes. Fans of this root may replace it with sweet potato.
- Vegetable oils: grapeseed oil, cottonseed oil , soybean oil, safflower oil , corn oil, sunflower oil, etc.
- Artificial sweeteners: sacharin, cyclamates, aspartame, sucralose & acesulfame potassium. Instead, use natural sweeteners, such as stevia.

Chapter 4: Gadgets & Cutlery

Although the Paleo diet follows the traditional caveman eating style where emphasis was on the unprocessed & the nutrient dense diet, a lot of the gadgets & cutlery used are modern. Choosing the kind of gadgets & kitchen equipment to buy may be tricky if you are not well-versed with them as a beginner. The list of items below may act as a guide to be used when shopping for kitchen utensils.

- **Knives**: The Paleo diet involves a lot of cutting of vegetables & meat. You'll require sharp knives that you may use for accurate cutting of the food. Go for a good knife that may last for a long time instead of a cheap one that might not give quality service. The blade of the knife should be extremely steady & strong with the handle well fastened.

- **Knife sharpener**: Due to constant use, the knife will be more likely to become blunt after use for a given period of time. A knife sharpener comes in handy for efficient use. Taking care of your knives will make them last much longer & be able to give you a quality service.

- **Kitchen shears**: Shears are helpful in trimming herbs or even cutting chicken. You can purchase a good quality of stainless steel that's made from high carbon. For easy cleaning, you can opt for shears that have separable blades.
- **Gloves**: To avoid the danger of being burnt by hot skillets and pots, you should at least have a pair of oven mitts. Towels work well, but having a pair of some heat-resistant gloves can be of great help.
- **Saucepan**: This high-sided pan is suitable for cooking foods like eggs or warming some leftover food. The Paleo diet does not entail cooking a lot of sauces, but a saucepan is quite handy. The stainless ones are suitable, although may be somewhat expensive.
- **Stock pot**: It is advisable to have at least one stock pot that can be used for boiling foods like meat, crabs or even making that homemade stock. Invest in one that's wide and capable of performing a variety of tasks.
- **Peeler**: This is kitchen equipment that you will require most of the time. You can invest in one that has a regular blade and makes work much easier. Peelers are not only used for peeling but can also serve as a gadget for

making shavings and ribbons of vegetables ideal for garnishing.

- **Cast Iron Skillet:** Cast iron skillets are ideal and are known to deliver quality service. The heavy and durable skillets are efficient and can withstand heat conduction with solid heat retention. Skillets are suitable for baking, searing and frying and once they are seasoned, they tend to develop that natural non-stick element. They are also suitable since they don't absorb the flavors from the food being cooked. Cast iron skillets are easy to clean as a stiff brush and hot water is enough for cleaning them.

- **Baking sheets**: Baking sheets are suitable for baking purposes. All you have to do is to line them with parchment or aluminum foil and it will be ready for use.

- **Spiralizer**: A spiralizer will provide you with fun ways of preparing your vegetables. You can turn the vegetables into noodles and is quite ideal for fun meals and snacks. You can spiralize a wide range of vegetables like sweet potatoes, apples, and zucchini amongst others.

- **Instant pot**: This programmable pressure cooker gives you the fun of preparing delicious meals with speed as you also save huge on energy. An instant pot provides the services of a slow cooker, rice cooker, yogurt maker amongst other cooking services.

- **Wire racks**: Wire racks are known for their versatility & you can use them to lift food items up over the fire when roasting.
- **Tongs**: Tongs are suitable for flipping food as you will not be using your hands for the work. All you need is a basic pair with wide scalloped pincers and you will be good. The locking tongs should be capable of giving you good grips when being used.
- **Immersion blender**: This gadget is suitable for cooking a wide range of foods like dressings, sauces, smoothies & dips. It's suitable for making foods like Paleo mayonnaise and the like.
- **Food processor**: This gadget is ideal for a variety of tasks like dicing, chopping, slicing & shredding all kinds of vegetables and fruits. A food processor will actually save you a lot of time and can be fun to work with.

Chapter 5: Recipes

Check out these fantastic paleo recipes.

Delightful Ultimate Paleo Almond Flour Muffins

I am interested!!

Ingredients:

- 3/4 tsp. baking soda
- 1/3 cup unsweetened pumpkin puree
- About 1 tsp. sea salt
- 3 large free-range eggs
- 2 tbsp. honey or maple syrup
- 2 tbsp. Melted coconut oil
- 2 cups almond meal or flour
- About 1.5 tsp. apple cider vinegar

Directions:

1. First of all, please make sure you have all the ingredients available. Preheat your oven to about 340 to 350°F.
2. Then prepare 10 muffin cups in a standard 12-cup muffin tin by lining then with paper liners.
3. This step is important. Whisk together almond flour, salt & baking soda (and any dried spices or herbs, if using).
4. Now wisk together eggs, extra virgin olive oil, vinegar, honey, and pumpkin in a small bowl

(whisk in any zest or extracts at this point, if using).

5. Next, please stir the wet ingredients into the dry mixture until well blended.
6. Almost there. One thing remains to be done now. Now divide the batter among the prepared cups & bake for about 15 to 20 minutes or maybe until the edges are golden brown & the centers set.
7. Finally transfer the tin to a cooling rack and let the muffins cool for at least 30 to 35 minutes before removing.

Servings: 10 to 12 Muffins

Total Time: 25 to 30 Minutes

Prep Time: 5 to 10 Minutes

Cooking Time: 15 to 20 Minutes

This never goes out of style.

Fantastic Feta Sweet Potato Jackets

Now be a legend!!

Ingredients:

- Pepper and salt to taste
- Crumbled feta cheese – 50g
- Finely sliced red onion – 1/4 piece
- Olive oil
- Finely chopped, deseeded fresh chili – about 1/2 teaspoon
- Roughly chopped fresh coriander – 1/2 tablespoon
- Lime halved juice – 2 tbsp.
- Plain yogurt – 3 grams
- Sweet potato – about 1.5

Directions:

1. First of all, please make sure you have all the ingredients available. Preheat the oven to about 390 to 400F.
2. Now cut sweet potato in half then place on a baking pan.
3. This step is important. Splash olive oil on the potato as you season with ground salt.
4. Place in the oven then bake for about 15 to 20 minutes or until tender.
5. Almost there. One thing remains to be done now. Then serve the sweet potato on a plate

& add red lime juice, chopped coriander & yogurt.

6. Finally add crumbled feta on top then add ground black pepper.

Prep time: 5 to 10 minutes

Cooking time: 15 to 20 minutes

Serves: 2 to 4

Simple yet fantastic!!

Nutritional Information:

Net carbs per serving – 27.2 g

Calories per serving – 303.2 g

Protein per serving – 9.7 g

Fat per serving – 17.9 g

Great Grilled Pork Chops with Stone Fruit Slaw

It is a brand new day…. Ever listened to this one!!

Ingredients:

For the Chops:

- 1 teaspoon ground paprika
- About 1.5 teaspoon sea salt
- 1 teaspoon ground cumin
- 1 teaspoon ground coriander
- 4 bone-in pork chops, about 1-1.5 inches thick

For the Slaw:

- Pinch sea salt
- About 1/2 teaspoon ground chipotle powder (or to taste, this amount will give it a good kick)
- 1 teaspoon lime juice
- About 1.5 teaspoon lime zest
- 1 pound assorted firm stone fruit (peaches, plums, apricots, etc.)

Directions:

1. First of all, please make sure you have all the ingredients available. Preheat your grill to medium-high heat & remove your pork chops from the fridge.

2. Then combine the teaspoon of cumin, salt, coriander and paprika in a small bowl & stir to combine

3. Divide the spice rub among the chops, making sure to coat both sides.

4. This step is important. Grill chops for about 5 to 10 minutes on each side, or until almost cooked through.

5. Now alternately, if you don't have a grill, Heat a large skillet over medium-high heat & add your preferred cooking fat (lard would be a good choice here) Sear the chops for about 5 to 8 minutes on each side, or maybe until almost cooked through.

6. Remove to a plate and cover loosely with foil, allowing them to rest for about 10 to 15 minutes.

7. Then meanwhile, prepare the slaw: Julienne fruit & place in a medium bowl.

8. Almost there. One thing remains to be done now. Mix in the chipotle powder, lime juice, lime zest, & a pinch of salt. Stir to combine.

9. Finally serve the chops topped with the slaw.

Serves: 3 to 4

Time to prepare: 30 to 40 minutes

 Awesome, isn't it?

Nutritional Information:

Calories: 231

Carbohydrates: 12.3g

Sugar: 9.8g

Fat: 9.5g

Saturated Fat: 3g

Protein: 23.2g

Happy Avocado Chicken Salad

Luxury tasty dish for you!!

Ingredients:

- 3 medium avocados
- A pinch of sea salt
- About 1.5 tbsp. avocado oil
- A pinch of freshly ground black pepper
- 1/2 red onion (Diced)
- 2 small tomatoes (Diced)
- Freshly squeezed lime juice from 1 lime
- About 1.5 tsp. chili powder
- 1 tsp. cumin
- 4 boneless and skinless chicken thighs

Directions:

1. First of all, please make sure you have all the ingredients available. Preheat your oven to about 340 to 350°F.
2. Now arrange chicken thighs in a baking dish & sprinkle with cumin, chili powder and sea salt.
3. Next, please drizzle with extra virgin olive oil & then bake for about 30 to 35 minutes or until the chicken is cooked through.

4. This step is important. Remove from oven & shred the chicken with two forks; set aside to cool.
5. Then mash avocado in a bowl until smooth & creamy.
6. Stir in lime juice, onion & tomato until well combined.
7. Now quickly remove from oven & then shred the chicken with two forks; set aside to cool.
8. Now mash avocado in a bowl until smooth and creamy.
9. Stir in lime juice, onion & tomato until well combined.
10. Almost there. One thing remains to be done now. Add the chicken & stir well.
11. Finally season with salt & pepper and serve immediately.

Servings: 4 to 6

Total Time: 45 to 50 Minutes

Prep Time: 45 to 50 Minutes

Cooking Time: 0 Minutes

Get ready to make it my way!!

Lucky Thai Coconut Soup

The best combo ever!!

Ingredients:

- 2 cups chicken stock
- Chopped cilantro for garnish
- 1 pound shrimp or chicken breast
- About 1.5 teaspoon sriracha
- About 1 inch piece of ginger, peeled & sliced into 1/8 inch rounds
- 1 tablespoon fish sauce
- 1 cup sliced mushrooms
- About 2.5 tablespoon lime juice
- 14 ounces full-fat coconut milk

Directions:

1. First of all, please make sure you have all the ingredients available. Peel and devein shrimp, if necessary, or if using chicken, remove connective tissues & cut into small pieces.
2. Now peel in slice ginger into 1/8-inch rounds.
3. Slice mushrooms.
4. This step is important. Add coconut milk, chicken stock & ginger to a pot & bring to boil over medium heat.

5.	Then reduce heat to simmer & add shrimp/chicken, mushrooms, lime juice, fish sauce & sriracha to the pot.
6.	Cook properly for less than 5 to 10 minutes, if using shrimp, & 5 to 10, if using chicken, or until cooked.
7.	Now meanwhile, chop cilantro.
8.	Almost there. One thing remains to be done now. Remove ginger from the soup (optional).
9.	Finally serve garnished with cilantro.

Something is new here!!

Vintage Basic Zucchini Noodle Bowl

A little work here but will be worth it.

Ingredients:

- 1 small sweet onion
- About 2.5 tablespoons grass-fed butter
- 2 crushed garlic cloves
- 2 large zucchinis

Directions:

1. First of all, please make sure you have all the ingredients available. Spiral the zucchini using a spiralizer. If you do not have one, slicing it very thin on a mandolin will work.
2. Now set aside.
3. Remove the outer layers of the onion & then slice thinly.
4. Heat butter in a saucepan over medium high heat until it melts.
5. This step is important. Then, toss in zucchini & onion and sauté until just cooked through.
6. Then this is where you can become creative.
7. Flavor the noodles anyway you wish with salt & pepper, or cayenne, or even lemon juice.

8. If topping with meat, cook the meat in another pan & then toss into this mixture once cooked through.

9. Now if adding fresh vegetables on top of it, toss right on in.

10.   Almost there. One thing remains to be done now. It can be flavored any way you like & added to anything you wish.

11.   Finally place everything into a bowl, top with anything else you want to top it with, & enjoy!

Try it…

Best Paleo Slow Cooker Pork Chili

This is different, isn't it?

Ingredients:

- 2 pounds pork shoulder
- Pinch of sea salt, fresh ground pepper, each
- About 2.5 onions (Chopped)
- 2 cans diced tomatoes
- 2 Tablespoons ground cumin
- 1 teaspoon black pepper
- 6 garlic cloves (Chopped)
- 3 Tablespoons dark cocoa powder
- 1 cup fresh chilies, finely chopped
- About 3.5 Tablespoons smoked paprika
- 4 pounds stewing beef
- 2 chipotle peppers (Chopped)

Garnish: cilantro

Directions:

1. First of all, please make sure you have all the ingredients available. Chop up the beef & pork into chunks.

2. Then add the onions, tomatoes, garlic, and chilies.
3. Stir until combined.
4. This step is important. Cover & cook properly on low for about 5 to 6 hours.
5. Now check meat doneness. Continue cooking if needed.
6. Almost there. One thing remains to be done now. Check at 30 to 35 minute intervals.
7. Finally serve in bowls. Garnish with cilantro.

Cooking Time: 5 to 6 hrs

Serving: 8 to 10

Yeah, this is a new variation.

Nutrition Facts (Per Serving):

787 Calories

41g Total Fat

14.4g Saturated Fat

0g Trans Fat

228mg Cholesterol

388mg Sodium

1671mg Potassium

36.1g Carbohydrates

13.9g Dietary Fiber

19.3g Sugars

71.1g Protein

Nostalgic Coconut vanilla ice cream

Classic, isn't it?

Ingredients:

Base:

- 4 egg yolks
- 1 can coconut milk
- About 4.5 tbsps real vanilla extract

Flavors:

- Citrus – lemon/orange/lime zest
- Coconut – 1/2 cup coconut flakes
- Berry – about 1 cup of any berries (Chopped)
- Honey – 3 tbsps raw honey
- Nut – 1/4 cup chopped nuts
- Mint – 1/2 cup finely chopped mint
- Chocolate – about 1/2 cup dark chocolate chips/flakes

Directions:

1. First of all, please make sure you have all the ingredients available. Pour some water in a pot, bring to a boil & reduce to a simmer.
2. Then place a heatproof bowl over it & pour in the milk.

3. Add vanilla extract & ingredients for the flavor you want, keep it hot, but make sure it doesn't come to a boil.
4. This step is important. Whisk the yolks in a bowl, add one ladleful of the milk mixture, whisking vigorously.
5. Now add 2 to 3 landlefuls, whisking constantly.
6. Add this mixture to the boil with hot milk, stir constantly to form a thick custard.
7. Then remove the bowl from the heat & let it cool.
8. Almost there. One thing remains to be done now. Pour the mixture in a baking dish & freeze for about 3.5 hours, stirring every 30 to 35 minutes.
9. Finally remove from the freezer for about 10 to 15 minutes before serving.

Cooking time: 25 to 30 minutes (3 hours to freeze)

Servings: 3 to 4 portions

Different yet fantastic in many ways.

Mighty Italian breakfast patties

Yeah, direct from the heaven; yeah?

Ingredients:

- Pinch cayenne and black pepper
- 1 tablespoon Italian spices
- 2 teaspoons dried parsley
- About 1/2 teaspoon turmeric
- 2 teaspoons granulated garlic
- 2 teaspoons granulated onion
- 1 teaspoon marjoram
- 1/2 teaspoon salt
- About 1.5 teaspoon paprika
- 2 tablespoons honey
- 1 teaspoon fennel seeds
- 1 teaspoon coconut oil
- 450g ground beef
- 1/2 teaspoon sage

Directions:

1. First of all, please make sure you have all the ingredients available. Next, please pre-heat a frying pan over medium heat, add coconut oil.

2. Then combine all the spices in a bowl & add to the ground beef.
3. Almost there. One thing remains to be done now. Now mix everything thoroughly with your hands, divide a mixture into parts & form round patties.
4. Finally fry each patty for about 2 to 5 minutes on one side, toss and fry for about 2 to 3 more minutes on the other.

It takes: 30 to 40 minutes

You get: 3 to 4 portions

What's so typical or different here?

King sized Delicious Beets and Carrots

Best combo ever… Don't you agree?

Ingredients:

- A pinch of sea salt
- 4 carrots, peeled and sliced
- About 2.5 tablespoons agave nectar
- 3 pounds red beets, peeled and cut into wedges
- About 2.5 teaspoons ginger, grated
- 3/4 cup pomegranate juice

Directions:

1. First of all, please make sure you have all the ingredients available. Put pomegranate juice in a pot & heat up over medium heat.
2. Now add a pinch of salt & the agave nectar, stir and cook properly for about 2 to 5 minutes.
3. Put beets and carrots in your slow cooker & ginger and stir gently.

4.   Almost there. One thing remains to be done now. Then add pomegranate juice, toss a bit, cover & cook properly on Low for about 5 to 6 hours.
5.   Finally divide beets and carrots between plates & serve warm or cold.

Preparation time: 10 to 15 minutes

Cooking time: 5 to 6 hours

Servings: 4 to 6

 Someone is definitely ready for this.

Nutritional information:

Fat 1

Protein 3

Fiber 2

Calories 100

Carbs 5

Crazy Turkey Scrambled Eggs

Good recipe!!

Ingredients:

- 200g pound minced turkey,
- About 1/2 tsp. sea salt
- 1 medium red bell pepper (Diced)
- 1/4 tsp. black pepper, freshly ground
- 1/2 medium yellow onion (Diced)
- 3 large free range eggs
- About 1/2 tsp. hot pepper sauce
- 1 tbsp. coconut oil

Directions:

1. First of all, please make sure you have all the ingredients available. Set a medium pan over medium high heat; add coconut oil & sauté onions until fragrant.
2. Now add turkey and red pepper; cook properly until turkey is done.
3. In the meantime, beat eggs in a bowl; stir in salt and pepper.
4. Pour the eggs into the pan with turkey, peppers, & onions.
5. Almost there. One thing remains to be done now. Then gently scramble the eggs until cooked.
6. Finally to serve, top with hot sauce.

Servings: 2 to 4

Total Time: 30 to 40 Minutes

Prep Time: 15 to 20 Minutes

Cooking Time: 15 to 20 Minutes

Lucky!!

Pinnacle Zucchini Pasta Pesto

Yes, this is famous!!

Ingredients:

- Sea salt
- Garlic walnut pesto roasted – 2/3 cup
- Fresh basil for garnishing
- Cherry tomatoes – about 1.5 cup
- Large zucchini – 2

Directions:

1. First of all, please make sure you have all the ingredients available. Now spiralize zucchini into noodles then salt & drain excess water.
2. Almost there. One thing remains to be done now. Then toss zucchini noodles with pesto & tomatoes until well combined.
3. Finally garnish the noodles with fresh basil.

Prep time: 20 to 25 minutes

Cooking time: 5 to 10

Serves: 2 to 3

Wow, that's cute!!

Nutritional Information:

Net carbs per serving – 29.5 g

Protein per serving – 8.8 g

Fat per serving – 16.2 g

Calories per serving – 292.7 g

Perfect Fennel and Brussels Sprouts Sirloin Rolls

Fresh start with something new!!

Ingredients:

<u>For the Filling:</u>

- About 1.5 tsp each of dried rosemary, sage and oregano
- 1/2 fennel bulb, roughly chopped
- 2 garlic cloves
- 1/2 cup Brussels sprouts, bottoms trimmed off and halved
- About 2 slices bacon, chopped into 4 or 5 large pieces

<u>Additional Ingredients:</u>

- 2 or 3 fennel fronds
- Salt and pepper, to taste
- About 1.5 tsp olive oil
- 2 cups Brussels sprouts (about 3/4 lb.), bottoms trimmed off and quartered
- 2 1/2 lb. sirloin steaks
- 1/2 fennel bulb, cut into thick slices

Directions:

1.   First of all, please make sure you have all the ingredients available. Preheat oven to about 360 to 370F.
2.   Then add all filling ingredients to a food processor.
3.   Process until it forms a thick paste.
4.   Now pound out steaks using a mallet until they are about 1/2 inch thick.
5.   This step is important. Next, please spread half of the filling on each steak.
6.   Now quickly roll steaks up, using a few toothpicks to secure.
7.   Next, please place sirloin rolls in a medium or large roasting pan & then sprinkle with salt & pepper.
8.   Now toss Brussels sprouts & fennel slices in a large bowl with olive oil, salt and pepper.
9.   Spread Brussels sprouts & fennel slices around sirloin rolls in the roasting pan.
10.   Then roast for about 35 to 40 minutes, until steak is cooked to desired level & vegetables begin to brown.
11.   If steak is done & veggies need to cook a bit longer, remove the steak from the pan & let it rest while you cook properly the veggies for an additional 5 to 10 minutes or so.

12.   Almost there. One thing remains to be done now. Let steak rest for about 5 to 10 minutes before slicing.
13.   Finally garnish with fennel fronds.

Serves: 3 to 4

Time to prepare: 40 to 50 minutes

Try this my way!!

Nutritional Information:

Calories: 641

Carbohydrates: 11.5g

Sugar: 1.6g

Fat: 23.4g

Saturated Fat: 8.2g

Protein: 92.7g

Dashing Paleo Chinese Chicken Salad

Baking does the trick!!

Ingredients:

- 1/2 cup cashews
- 1/2 tsp. sea salt
- About 2.5 tbsp. white sesame seeds
- 2 tbsp. black sesame seeds
- 1/4 cup tamari or regular soy sauce
- 1/2 cup chopped cilantro
- 1 head of Napa cabbage, thinly chopped
- 2 bags shredded carrots
- 1/4 cup white wine vinegar
- 5 chopped green onions, green, and white parts
- About 1.5 tsp. Sirach
- 1 tsp. spicy chili oil
- 3 tbsp. finely minced ginger
- 1 tbsp. toasted sesame oil
- 2 tbsp. hoisin sauce
- 1 rotisserie chicken, torn into shreds
- 3 tbsp. extra virgin olive oil

Directions:

1. First of all, please make sure you have all the ingredients available. Make the dress: In a mason jar with a lid, mix extra virgin olive

oil, minced garlic, Sirach, vinegar, tamari, hoisin sauce, chili oil, toasted sesame oil, chopped green onions & sea salt.
2. Then secure the lid & shake to mix well; set aside.
3. Almost there. One thing remains to be done now. Now in a large plastic bag, combine shredded chicken, chopped cabbage, sesame seeds, shredded carrots, cilantro, cashews, & enough dressing; shake well to mix.
4. Finally serve the salad into bowls & enjoy!

Servings: 4 to 6

Total Time: 20 to 30 Minutes

Prep Time: 20 to 25 Minutes

Cooking Time: 5 to 10 Minutes

I don't know about you, but I include this one everytime I get a chance.

Reliable Beef Zoodle Soup

I repeat… Try it if you want to. No regrets. Right!!

Ingredients:

- About 11 to 12 ounces boneless beef sirloin steak, thinly sliced across the grain
- 1 small onion, halved & thinly sliced
- 5 to 6 ounces fresh shiitake mushrooms, stemmed and sliced
- About 2 medium zucchini
- 2 cloves garlic, minced
- About 2.5 teaspoons minced fresh ginger
- 1 teaspoon sea salt
- 5 cups beef bone broth
- 2 tablespoons coconut aminos
- About 2.5 teaspoons fish sauce
- 1 tablespoon coconut oil

Toppings:

- Lime wedges
- Fresh cilantro leaves
- Sliced jalapeño
- Sliced green onion
- Fresh basil leaves

Directions:

1. First of all, please make sure you have all the ingredients available. Halve and thinly

slice the onion, stem & slice mushrooms, and mince garlic & fresh ginger.

2. Now add coconut oil to a large pot & heat it over medium heat.

3. Add onion to the pot and cook properly for about 2 to 5 minutes, stirring, until softened.

4. This step is important. Add the mushrooms & cook properly for another 2 minutes, continuing to stir once in a while.

5. Add the garlic and ginger & cook properly or 30 to 40 seconds or until aromatic.

6. Then pour in beef bone broth.

7. Add coconut aminos, fish sauce, & salt and bring to a boil then simmer on medium-low, uncovered, for about 5 to 10 minutes.

8. Now with the help of a spiralizer or maybe julienne peeler cut the zucchini lengthwise into thin strands.

9. Now thinly slice across the grain the steak (freeze for 15 to 20 minutes to make it easier).

10. Add zucchini noodles to the pot & cook properly for about 2 minutes, until tender.

11. Almost there. One thing remains to be done now. Add steak slice & cook properly for about 30 to 60 seconds.

12.	Finally serve in bowl topped with fresh basil leaves, green onion, cilantro leaves, jalapeno slices or lemon wedges.

Why not??

Charming Don't Down The Greats Salad

Leave a mark!!

Ingredients:

- 1/2 cup organic salad dressing (make sure it has no added sugars, such as fructose, and no dairy incorporated)
- About 1 to 2 chicken breasts
- Crumbled bacon (optional)
- About 2.5 tablespoons butter (can be substituted for coconut oil)
- Components for preferred salad base

Directions:

1. First of all, please make sure you have all the ingredients available. Heat butter (or coconut oil) over medium high heat in a saucepan.
2. Now add sliced chicken breasts & cook properly until no pink is showing in the middle. Set aside.

3. Almost there. One thing remains to be done now. Then assemble all the components necessary for your preferred salad in a bowl.
4. Finally put the chicken on top of the salad, sprinkle with crumbled bacon (optional), & top with your salad dressing of choice!

Spice up!!

Energetic Paleo Meat & Veggies Chili

What do you think? ?

Ingredients:

- About 2.5 Tablespoons olive oil
- 15 ounce can diced tomatoes
- 2 garlic cloves (Chopped)
- 2 large zucchini (Diced)
- 1 celery stalk (Chopped)
- 1 large onion (Diced)
- 1 carrot (Diced)
- 15 ounce can tomato sauce
- About 2.5 Tablespoons chili powder
- 1 teaspoon oregano
- 1 teaspoon ground cumin
- 11/2 pounds lean ground beef
- 1/4 teaspoon cayenne pepper (Optional)

Garnish: chopped parsley

Directions:

1. First of all, please make sure you have all the ingredients available. Next, please place all the ingredients in your slow cooker.

2. Then cover and cook properly on low for about 5 to 6 hours, until meat is cooked & vegetables are fork tender.
3. Almost there. One thing remains to be done now. Now serve hot.
4. Finally side with rice or bread.

Cooking Time: 4 to 6 hrs

Serving: 6 to 8

What makes this the best? Check it out for yourself!!

Nutrition Facts (Per Serving):

7.9g Saturated Fat

0g Trans Fat

12.3g Sugars

98.5g Protein

279mg Cholesterol

599mg Sodium

721 Calories

2185mg Potassium

23.7g Total Fat

25.3g Carbohydrates

6.7g Dietary Fiber

Funny BBQ grilled peaches with cinnamon

Just got better!!

Ingredients:

- About 2.5 tbsps coconut oil
- 4 peaches
- Ground cinnamon to taste

Directions:

1. First of all, please make sure you have all the ingredients available. Preheat the BBQ grill to medium-low.
2. Now halve and pit the peaches, & brush them with coconut oil from both sides.
3. Almost there. One thing remains to be done now. Then place on the grill & cook properly for about 4.5 minutes per side.
4. Sprinkle with cinnamon & serve.

Cooking time: 10 to 15 minutes

Servings: 4 to 6 portions

Got the idea!!

Scrumptious Sausage veggie hash

Relax and enjoy this recipe!!

Ingredients:

- 3 zucchinis
- About 1.5 tablespoon coconut oil
- 2 sweet potatoes
- 1/2 avocado
- About 1.5 onion
- 450g breakfast sausage

Directions:

1. First of all, please make sure you have all the ingredients available. Pre-heat a large frying pan over medium-high heat, add coconut oil.
2. Now wash vegetables, dry them with paper towels, peel them.
3. Dice onions & sweet potatoes, slice zucchini and avocado.
4. This step is important. Slice breakfast sausage & fry it for about 5 to 10 minutes, remove from the pan.
5. Then place diced onion, fry for about 2 minutes.
6. Almost there. One thing remains to be done now. Add diced sweet potatoes to onion,

cover with the lid and cook properly for about 10 to 15 minutes.

7. Finally add sliced zucchini & fry for about 5 to 10 more minutes, return fried sausages to a pan & combine the ingredients well.

It takes: 30 to 35 minutes

You get: 4 to 5 portions

Try this one if you're hungry!!

Astonishing Special Acorn Squash and Cranberry Sauce

Make me remember the good old days!!

Ingredients:

- 2 acorn squash, peeled and cut into medium wedges
- Black pepper to the taste
- 16 ounces canned cranberry sauce, unsweetened
- A pinch of sea salt
- About 1/2 teaspoon cinnamon, ground
- 1/4-cup raisins

Directions:

1. First of all, please make sure you have all the ingredients available. Now place acorn pieces in your slow cooker, add cinnamon, cranberry sauce, raisins, salt & pepper, stir, cover and cook properly on Low for about 6 to 7 hours.
2. Finally divide between plates & serve hot as a Paleo side.

Preparation time: 10 to 15 minutes

Cooking time: 5 to 7 hours

Servings: 4 to 6

Luxury in its own class!!

Nutritional information:

Protein 2

Fat 3

Carbs 10

Fiber 3

Calories 230

Excellent Tapioca Crêpes

Healthy is a new trend these days!! ? Always I guess...

Ingredients:

- 1 cup full fat coconut milk
- About 1/2 tsp. sea salt
- 1 cup tapioca flour
- Toppings of choice- for crepes, (I prefer almond butter and berries, but you can also mix it up with cinnamon, applesauce, sautéed veggies, etc.)
- 1 large free range egg

Directions:

1. First of all, please make sure you have all the ingredients available. In a medium bowl, please mix together all the ingredients.
2. Then set a skillet over medium heat & add 1/3 cup of the mixture when hot, tilting the skillet to spread out the batter.
3. Almost there. One thing remains to be done now. Now cook both sides for about 2 to 5 minutes or until lightly browned.
4. Finally serve warm topped with desired ingredients.

Servings: 2 to 4

Total Time: 35 to 40 Minutes

Prep Time: 10 to 15 Minutes

Cooking Time: 25 to 30 Minutes

Stunner!!

Legendary Paleo Fish and Chips

Iconic recipe of my list!!

Ingredients:

<u>For batter:</u>

- Coconut oil – 1 cup
- Sea salt – about 1.5 teaspoon
- Almond flour – 1 cup
- Coconut milk – 1/2 cup
- Eggs (organic or soy free eggs) – 2
- Wild caught cod – 1 lb

<u>For sweet potato chips:</u>

- Coconut oil – 3 cups
- Sea salt – about 2.5 tsp
- Pepper – 1 tbsp.
- Medium Sweet Potatoes – 5

Directions:

1. First of all, please make sure you have all the ingredients available. Combine sea salt, almond flour, coconut milk & eggs into a food processor then mix well
2. Then cut the cod into small strips
3. This step is important. Heat coconut oil, batter the cod, then fry until golden brown.

4. Peel sweet potatoes then slice into thin strips.
5. Now add salt and pepper to the sliced potatoes & fry using coconut oil until brown.
6. Almost there. One thing remains to be done now. Set it on a paper towel to soak the grease.
7. Finally serve together with the fish then enjoy.

Prep time: 10 to 15 minutes

Cooking time: 20 to 25

Serves: 2 to 3

Well it is a Grandma's recipe!!

Nutritional Information:

Net carbs per serving – 20 g

Protein per serving – 33 g

Fat per serving – 13 g

Calories per serving – 338 g

Awesome Paleo Spaghetti Squash & Meatballs

Happiness has finally arrived!!

Ingredients:

- Italian seasoning (Oregano, Basil, Thyme) to taste, I used about 2 tsp
- 1 pound of ground Italian sausage.
- 1 can of tomato sauce, I used a 14 ounce can.
- About 2.5 tbsp. of olive oil.
- 2 tbsp. of hot pepper relish (optional).
- 4 to 6 cloves of garlic, whole.
- About 1.5 medium spaghetti squash.

Directions:

1. First of all, please make sure you have all the ingredients available. Make sure you use a large 6 quart slow cooker for this recipe.
2. Now dump your tomato sauce, garlic, olive oil, hot pepper relish and Italian seasoning into your slow cooker & stir well.
3. This step is important. Next, please cut your squash in half & scoop out the seeds.
4. Place your 2 squash halves face down into your slow cooker.

5. Then roll your ground sausage into meatballs, then fit as many as you can in the sauce around the squash.

6. I was able to work in about a half pound worth.

7. Almost there. One thing remains to be done now. Cook properly on High for about 3.5 hours or cook on low for about 5.5 hours.

8. Finally use a large fork to pull the "spaghetti" out of your squash, then top with your meatballs & sauce.

Serves: 3 to 4

Time to prepare: 5 hours 30 to 40 minutes (5 hours in crock pot)

Whenever you want a great recipe!!

Nutritional Information:

Calories: 473

Carbohydrates: 12.7g

Sugar: 5.1g

Fat: 35.4g

Saturated Fat: 10.2g

Protein: 21.3g

Quick Seared Tuna Nicosia Salad

How is it? Only one way to find out…

Ingredients:

- 2 ounces trimmed French green beans
- 1 tsp. water
- About 2.5 tsp. capers
- 1/4 tsp. sea salt
- 1 tbsp. extra-virgin olive oil
- 1/2 garlic clove (Minced)
- Fresh cracked black pepper
- 1/4 tsp. maple syrup
- About 1.5 tsp. Dijon mustard
- 1 tbsp. fresh lemon juice
- Olive oil cooking spray
- 8-ounce tuna steak
- 2 hard-boiled eggs (Sliced)
- 4 radishes, sliced thin
- 1/4 cup fresh basil leaves
- 2 small cucumbers, thinly sliced crosswise
- About 1/2 red onion, thinly sliced
- 2 cups petite lettuce leaves
- 1/2 cup cherry tomatoes, halved

Directions:

1. First of all, please make sure you have all the ingredients available. Now please bring a

pot of water to a gentle boil; add beans & boil for about 2 to 5 minutes or until crisp-tender and bright green.

2. Now drain the beans & plunge into iced water; drain and set aside.

3. Arrange the lettuce, basil, cucumbers, onion, tomatoes, green beans, eggs, and radishes evenly between 2 serving plates.

4. This step is important. Set a skillet over medium high heat & coat with olive oil cooking spray.

5. Then season tuna with sea salt & pepper and add to the pan; cook for about 3 to 6 minutes per side or maybe until browned.

6. Cut cooked tuna across the grain & arrange over veggies.

7. Almost there. One thing remains to be done now. Make the dressing: mix together lemon juice with other dressing ingredients in a jar & secure the lid; shake until well blended.

8. Now finally drizzle the dressing over the salad and serve.

Servings: 2 to 4

Total Time: 30 to 40 Minutes

Prep Time: 25 to 30 Minutes

Cooking Time: 5 to 10 Minutes

I can eat them all day!!

Wonderful Paleo Olive Pizza

Different take on this one…

Ingredients:

- Watercress (can substitute for spinach)
- 3 eggs, beaten
- 1 cup water
- About 3.5 tablespoons organic Italian seasonings and spices
- 2 cups grass-fed organic mozzarella cheese
- 1/2 cup organic tomato sauce
- About 1 tablespoon coconut oil
- Pinch of salt
- Fresh olives, pitted and sliced
- 1/2 cup coconut flour

Directions:

1. First of all, please make sure you have all the ingredients available. Preheat oven to about 390 to 400 degrees.
2. Now sift the flour into a bowl & add the eggs, salt, and water. Incorporate well.

3. Heat your cast iron skillet over high heat until very hot.
4. Place coconut oil into pan & let it melt.
5. This step is important. Pour in half of the crust mixture & let it cook properly until the top begins to bubble.
6. Then once it bubbles, flip to cook the other side.
7. Once the other side begins to bubble, add desired sauce & toppings and transfer the entire thing to a plate.
8. Now repeat process to make another pizza.
9. Almost there. One thing remains to be done now. Put the pizzas in the oven for about 5 to 10 minutes until the crust begins to firm.
10. Finally pull them out & enjoy!

Grandfather of Recipes!!

Elegant Slow Cooker Thai Beef Stew

I am actually popular among my friends for eating this one a lot.

Ingredients:

- About 2.5 Tablespoons coconut oil (for searing beef)
- 1 cup peeled jicama
- 2 garlic cloves (Minced)
- 2 cups broccoli (Diced)
- 1 medium yellow onion (Sliced)
- 13.5 ounce can coconut milk, full fat
- 2 cups carrots (Diced)
- 1 inch piece ginger, peeled and minced
- 1/3 cup tomato paste
- About 2.5 teaspoons fresh lime juice
- 2 Tablespoon fish sauce
- 1/2 cup Thai red curry paste
- 1 teaspoon sea salt
- 3 pounds stewing beef

Directions:

1. First of all, please make sure you have all the ingredients available. Cooked or

uncooked, place the chunks of beef in the crock pot.

2.   Now add the other ingredients (not the oil, only use that for searing) to the crock pot.
3.   This step is important. Stir until combined.
4.   Then cover & cook properly on low for about 4 to 5 hours, until meat is done.
5.   Almost there. One thing remains to be done now. Serve warm.
6.   Finally side with rice & pita bread/naan.

Cooking Time: 4 to 5 hrs

Serving: 6 to 8

So, what's your opinion?

Nutrition Facts (Per Serving):

0g Trans Fat

152mg Cholesterol

54.3g Protein

1757mg Sodium

1035mg Potassium

5.1g Sugars

15.1g Carbohydrates

540 Calories

27.5g Total Fat

16.6g Saturated Fat

2.9g Dietary Fiber

Rich Almond milk custard

Yeah, you can make it in your free time…

Ingredients:

- 2 cups unsweetened almond milk
- Cinnamon and nutmeg to taste
- About 1/2 cup honey
- Hot water
- About 2.5 tsp vanilla extract
- 5 eggs

Directions:

1. First of all, please make sure you have all the ingredients available. Preheat oven to about 310 to 320 F.
2. Then pour milk & honey in a saucepan, gently bring to a simmer and remove from the heat.
3. Whisk eggs with the vanilla extract in a bowl until well combined.
4. Slowly whisk the milk, be careful not to cook the eggs.
5. This step is important. Pour the mixture in individual ramequins & place them in a baking dish.
6. Now pour in it warm water, up to the same level as the custard in the ramequins.

7. Place the dish in the oven & cook properly for about 35 to 40 minutes, until edges are set.
8. Almost there. One thing remains to be done now. Then remove from the oven, cool for some time & put in the fridge for about 2.5 hours.
9. Finally sprinkle with cinnamon & nutmeg to taste & serve.

Cooking time: 2 to 3 hours

Servings: 5 to 6 portions

Supremacy defined!!

Titanic Sweet potato cookies

A simple recipe which you will like.

Ingredients:

- 150g almond flour
- About 1 teaspoon baking powder
- 70g walnuts
- 1 tablespoon coconut oil
- 60ml coconut milk
- 1 egg
- About 1.5 tablespoon cinnamon
- 2 tablespoons maple syrup
- 3 sweet potatoes

Directions:

1. First of all, please make sure you have all the ingredients available. Pre-heat a pan, pour water & bring to a boil.
2. Now peel sweet potatoes, transfer them to a boiling water & cook properly for about 20 to 25 minutes.
3. Mash when cooked.
4. This step is important. Pre-heat an oven over medium-high heat, cover the baking tray with the parchment, grease it with coconut oil.
5. Then whisk eggs, mix them with maple syrup & coconut milk.

6. Stir almond flour, cinnamon & baking powder in the mixture, mix thoroughly.
7. Now add mashed sweet potatoes, combine well.
8. Almost there. One thing remains to be done now. Place a spoonful of the mixture on the baking tray until there is no mixture left.
9. Finally bake for about 20 to 25 minutes.

It takes: 45 to 50 minutes

You get: 2 to 4 portions

A fine recipe, it just works.

Tasty Crazy Eggplant Delight

Yummy, definitely yummy.

Ingredients:

- 1 tablespoon olive oil
- A handful cilantro (Chopped)
- 2 garlic cloves (Minced)
- About 1.5 teaspoon cumin, ground
- 2 carrots (Chopped)
- 1 yellow onion (Chopped)
- A pinch of cayenne pepper
- 10 ounces canned tomatoes, roughly chopped
- About 1.5 tablespoon ras all hanout
- 1 eggplant, roughly chopped

Directions:

1. First of all, please make sure you have all the ingredients available. Then put the oil in your slow cooker.
2. Add eggplant, garlic, tomatoes, carrots, onion, cumin, ras eh hanout and cayenne.

3. Almost there. One thing remains to be done now. Now toss everything, cover & cook properly on Low for about 5 to 6 hours.
4. Finally sprinkle cilantro on top, divide between plates & serve with a tasty pork steak.

Preparation time: 10 to 15 minutes

Cooking time: 5 to 6 hours

Servings: 4 to 6

Don't wait, eat it!!

Nutritional information:

Fat 4

Carbs 10

Protein 3

Fiber 2

Calories 120

Yummy Thick & Creamy Strawberry Banana Shake

Just make it once and you will keep making it!!

Ingredients:

- 1/2 cup frozen strawberries
- About 1 tsp. vanilla extract
- 2/3 cup almond milk
- 1 scoop vanilla protein powder (Optional)
- 1 banana, frozen
- 1/2 cup orange juice
- About 1 tbsp. ground chia seeds

Directions:

1. Please combine all ingredients in a blender & blend until very smooth. There you go!!

Servings: 1 to 2

Total Time: 5 to 10 Minutes

Prep Time: 5 to 10 Minutes

I've always loved them. Plus they can be eaten anytime!!

Unique Beef Liver with Onions

Good luck!!

Ingredients:

- Sea salt
- Large sweet onion – 1
- Lard or butter – about 3.5 tablespoons
- Sage and fresh thyme
- Beef liver slices – 3/4 slices (previously marinated)

Directions:

1. First of all, please make sure you have all the ingredients available. Thinly slice the onions then melt lard in a nonstick pan & place over slow flame.
2. Then add the finely chopped herbs & onions then stir for about 10 to 15 minutes until translucent.
3. Remove the onions & place on a plate then set aside & keep warm.
4. This step is important. Increase the flame as you add one more tablespoon of lard.
5. Now add the liver once the lard is hot.
6. Sauté until browned on the bottom or for about 2 to 5 minutes and flip it over.

7. Almost there. One thing remains to be done now. Now quickly add the onions back to the pan as you lower the flame.
8. Finally allow it to cook properly for about 2 to 5 more minutes until pink inside.

Prep time: 5 to 10 minutes

Cooking time: 15 to 20 minutes

Serves: 4 to 5

Oh yeah!!

Nutritional Information:

Net carbs per serving – 35 g

Protein per serving – 41 g

Fat per serving – 18.3 g

Calories per serving – 468 g

Ultimate Paleo Pulled Pork Sliders

Stupidly simple…

Ingredients:

- Large pork roast
- Juice of 1 lemon
- 1 large onion (Sliced)
- 3 minced garlic cloves
- Juice of 1 lime
- 2 tsp cumin
- 2 tsp chili powder
- 1 tsp pepper
- 2 tsp sea salt
- 2 tsp oregano
- 1 tsp paprika
- 1/2 tsp cayenne pepper
- 1/2 tsp cinnamon
- Pulled Pork

Directions:

1. First of all, please make sure you have all the ingredients available. Stir together the spices and rub all over the roast.
2. Then lay the onion slices down on the bottom of the slow cooker, and squeeze half of the fruit juices in.
3. Put the roast in the crockpot and squeeze the remaining lime and lemon juice over it.

4.   Almost there. One thing remains to be done now. Now cook properly on low overnight or throughout the day about 8 hours (you really can't overcook it to be honest).

5.   Finally when done, shred it with two forks until it's completely 'pulled'.

Ingredients:

- Dash of sea salt
- 1 large sweet potato (try to go for a nice evenly round one, remember the diameter will be the size of your sliders)
- About 1/2 tsp paprika
- 2 tbsp. coconut oil
- The "Buns"
- About 1/2 tsp cumin

Directions:

1.   First of all, please make sure you have all the ingredients available. Now quickly slice the sweet potato into 1/4" thick rounds. Lay them out on a parchment paper-lined cookie sheet.

2.	Then quickly brush each slice with coconut oil & sprinkle with the spices, then flip and do the same on the other side.
3.	This step is important. Bake at about 410 to 420 degrees Fahrenheit for about 30 to 35 minutes until golden brown on the outside & cooked all the way through, flipping halfway through.
4.	Now you may need to crank it up to 450.
5.	Almost there. One thing remains to be done now. Top a patty with pulled pork, & add any other toppings or sauces you'd
6.	Finally finish with the top patty & enjoy.

Serves: 3 to 4

Time to prepare: 8 hours 30 to 40 minutes (8 hours cooking in crock pot)

Be unique, be extraordinary…

Nutritional Information:

Carbohydrates: 16.2g

Protein: 14.2g

Sugar: 4.8g

Saturated Fat: 7.4g

Fat: 11.6g

Calories: 220

Iconic Tomato & Tuna Burgers

Something is special!!

Ingredients:

- 1 cup tuna, drained, rinsed
- A pinch of sea salt
- About 2.5 tbsp. Tomato paste
- A pinch of freshly ground black pepper
- 1 egg
- 1 small finely chopped red onion
- 1 garlic clove, crushed
- 1 small finely chopped red chili
- About 1.5 tbsp. coconut flour

Optional for serving

- Fresh coriander (cilantro)
- Lettuce
- Avocado
- Extra chili

Directions:

1. First of all, please make sure you have all the ingredients available. Preheat your oven to about 340 to 350°F.
2. Then line a baking tray with parchment paper; set aside.
3. This step is important. Combine burger ingredients in a bowl & stir to mix well.

4. Carefully roll and flatten tuna mixture with your hands into 6, equal sized patties & arrange them on the mined baking tray.
5. Almost there. One thing remains to be done now. Now bake for about 10 to 15 minutes or until cooked through.
6. Finally to serve, place each burger into a lettuce leaf & top with sliced avocado, & sprinkle with extra slices of chili and fresh coriander.

Servings: 4 to 6 Burgers

Total Time: 55 to 60 Minutes

Prep Time: 15 to 20 Minutes

Cooking Time: 40 to 50 Minutes

If you're a legend, then make this one.

Awesome Thai Vegetable Soup

Being lucky is definitely better.

Ingredients:

- 1 onion, finely chopped
- 1/2 cup cilantro (Minced)
- About 2 cups sliced shiitake mushrooms, trim off bottom of stems
- About 1/2 teaspoon sea salt
- 1 quart pacific foods organic vegetable broth
- 1 cup full fat coconut milk
- 2 tablespoons lime juice, freshly squeezed
- 1 head broccoli, trimmed and chopped
- About 1.5 tablespoon fresh ginger root (Minced)
- 2 tablespoons olive oil

Directions:

1. First of all, please make sure you have all the ingredients available. Finely chop onion.
2. Now cut off the bottom of stems from the mushrooms & slice the mushrooms.
3. Trim and chop broccoli & mince ginger root.

4.   Add oil to a large saucepan & heat over medium heat.

5.   This step is important. Add onion to the saucepan & cook, stirring often, for about 10 to 15 minutes or until softened.

6.   Then add mushrooms & cook properly for another 5 to 10 minutes.

7.   Next, please pour in broth & then coconut milk & bring to simmer, then reduce heat to medium.

8.   Add broccoli and ginger and cook properly for about 2 to 5 minutes, until the broccoli is bright green.

9.   Almost there. One thing remains to be done now. Now add lime juice & salt. Chop cilantro.

10.   Finally serve the soup in bowls, garnished with cilantro.

Mystery is unveiled!!

Super Vegetable Stir Fry With Peppers And Green Beans

The speed matters…

Ingredients:

- Pinch of red pepper flakes
- 1 small red onion
- 3 cloves garlic
- About 1/2 teaspoon ginger powder
- Pinch of salt
- 1 cup broccoli florets
- 2 tablespoons white cooking wine
- 1/2 julienned red pepper
- 1/2 julienned yellow pepper
- About 2.5 tablespoons soy sauce
- 1/2 cup fresh green beans
- 1 small carrot, sliced
- 5 fresh mushrooms
- 2 tablespoons grass-fed butter

Directions:

1. First of all, please make sure you have all the ingredients available. Heat a wok or pan

over medium high heat & melt butter into pan.

2. Now slice and dice vegetables accordingly, & add them to the wok or pan.
3. Add a little bit of salt.
4. This step is important. Stir fry all vegetables together for about 5 to 10 minutes.
5. Then gently turn temperature down to low and let sit.
6. In a small bowl, combine all of your wet ingredients, plus the ginger powder & red pepper flakes.
7. Almost there. One thing remains to be done now. Add this mixture to the vegetables & toss them until lightly coated.
8. Finally add to serving dish & enjoy!

Be super

Delightful Crock Pot Beef Stroganoff

Deserved!!

Ingredients:

- 2 teaspoons paprika
- Pinch of sea salt, fresh ground pepper, each
- About 2.5 teaspoons red wine vinegar
- 1/3 cup coconut cream
- 1 teaspoon garlic powder
- 1/2 cup mushrooms (Sliced)
- 1 teaspoon onion powder
- About 1.5 teaspoon thyme
- 2 pounds stewing beef
- 1/2 medium white onion (Sliced)

Directions:

1. First of all, please make sure you have all the ingredients available. Place the mushrooms & onions in the bottom of the crock pot.
2. Now place the meat, cooked or uncooked, on top of the vegetables.
3. Pour the seasoning over the meat.

4. This step is important. Pour the red wine vinegar in the crock pot.

5. Then cover & cook properly on low for about 4 to 5 hours.

6. Once the meat is cooked, turn the crock pot to high, add the cream.

7. Now stir until it thickens the sauce.

8. Almost there. One thing remains to be done now. Serve warm.

9. Finally side with noodles, rice, or naan bread.

Cooking Time: 4 to 5 hrs

Serving: 6 to 8

Long way to go...

Nutrition Facts (Per Serving):

6.4g Saturated Fat

47.7g Protein

0g Trans Fat

135mg Cholesterol

880mg Sodium

1.8g Sugars

808mg Potassium

4.1g Carbohydrates

330 Calories

12.8g Total Fat

1.3g Dietary Fiber

Fantastic Pumpkin pie

Cooking level infinite….

Ingredients:

Crust:

- 1/2 cup hazelnuts
- 1 pinch of sea salt
- 1 cup pecans
- About 4.5 tbsps butter/coconut oil (room temperature)

Filling:

- 2 eggs
- 1/4 tsp fresh grated ginger
- 1/2 cup coconut milk
- About 1/2 tsp ground cloves
- 1/2 cup raw honey
- 1 can fresh/canned pumpkin puree
- 2 tsp cinnamon

Directions:

1. First of all, please make sure you have all the ingredients available. Preheat oven to about 340 to 350 F.
2. Then grind the nuts in a food processor to almost nut flour.

3. This step is important. Mix them with the butter or coconut oil in a bowl.
4. Spread the mixture in a pie pan & bake for about 10 to 15 minutes.
5. Almost there. One thing remains to be done now. Now mix all the ingredients for the filling.
6. Finally add the mixture evenly on the bakes crust & put back in the oven for about 40 to 45 minutes.

Cooking time: 1 to 2 hour

Servings: 4 to 5 portions

Uber fantastic!!

Great Pumpkin pancakes

For those who are not ordinary, try this one.

Ingredients:

- 1/2 cup canned pumpkin
- 2 tbsps butter or coconut oil
- About 1.5 tsp pure vanilla extract
- 1/4 tsp baking soda
- 2 tbsps pure maple syrup (optional)
- About 1.5 tsp cinnamon
- 1 tsp pumpkin pie spice
- 4 eggs

Directions:

1. First of all, please make sure you have all the ingredients available. Whisk the eggs, pure vanilla extract, canned pumpkin, and pure maple syrup & mix the ingredients.
2. Then add the pumpkin pie spice, cinnamon, & baking soda.
3. Mix 2 tsp of melted butter into the batter.
4. This step is important. Put some butter in the skillet.
5. Now start frying as the butter melts.
6. Flip the pancakes once, when they are ready.

7. Almost there. One thing remains to be done now. Continue to cook properly until both sides are crispy and golden.
8. Finally serve with grass-fed butter & cinnamon or sliced bananas.

It takes: 20 to 30 minutes

You get: 6 to 8 small pancakes

Be amazed ?

Happy Tasty Zucchini

Wow, just wow!!

Ingredients:

- About 1.5 teaspoon Italian seasoning
- 1/4 cup pork rinds, crushed
- Black pepper to the taste
- 2 cups yellow squash, peeled and cut into wedges
- A pinch of sea salt
- About 1.5 teaspoon garlic powder
- 2 cups zucchinis (Sliced)
- 2 tablespoons olive oil

Directions:

1. First of all, please make sure you have all the ingredients available. Now put the oil in your slow cooker.
2. Almost there. One thing remains to be done now. Then add zucchini and squash pieces, Italian seasoning, black pepper, salt and garlic powder, toss well, cover &

cook properly on Low for about 5 to 6 hours.

3. Finally divide between plates & serve with pork rind sprinkled on top.

Preparation time: 10 to 15 minutes

Cooking time: 5 to 6 hours

Servings: 6 to 8

Show time!!

Nutritional information:

Fat 2

Carbs 8

Fiber 4

Calories 100

Protein 5

Lucky Pumpkin and Banana Smoothie

Feast for you!!

Ingredients:

- 1 heaping scoop vanilla protein powder (Optional)
- 1 cup almond milk
- 1 frozen banana
- 1/3 cup pumpkin puree
- About 1.5 tbsp. honey or maple syrup

Directions:

1. First of all, please make sure you have all the ingredients available. Now combine all ingredients in a blender & blend until very smooth.

Servings: 2 to 4

Total Time: 5 to 10 Minutes

Prep Time: 5 to 10 Minutes

Being super is a matter of recipe… ?

Vintage Gluten Free Banana Nut Muffins

Being a legend.

Ingredients:

- Organic vanilla extract – 4
- Chopped nuts – 1/2 cup
- Organic eggs (Pasture raised) – 4
- Blanched almond flour – 3 cups
- Pure maple syrup – about 1.5 tablespoon
- Coconut oil – 6 tablespoons
- Peeled ripe bananas – 3

Directions:

1. First of all, please make sure you have all the ingredients available. Preheat the oven to about 310 to 320F.
2. Then in a glass bowl mash the peeled bananas using a potato masher or fork until fairly smooth.
3. Add vanilla extract, maple syrup & eggs then mix well.
4. This step is important. Add coconut oil and mix; slowly add the chopped nuts, almond flour & then mix well.
5. Now place the mixture into parchment muffin cups in a muffin tin & smooth the top.
6. Almost there. One thing remains to be done now. Bake the mixture for about 25 to 30

minutes or until the top begins to brown slightly.

7. Finally serve with fresh butter.

Prep time: 5 to 10 minutes

Cooking time: 20 to 25

Serves: 3 to 4

When you're fantastic, this is best!!

Nutritional Information:

Net carbs per serving – 23.2 g

Calories per serving – 184.3 g

Protein per serving – 3.8 g

Fat per serving – 9.2 g

Best Paleo Crockpot Jambalaya Soup

Being rich is a plus point ?

Ingredients:

- About 1/4 cup Frank's Red Hot (or hot sauce of your choice)
- 4 peppers – any color you want (Chopped)
- 1 large onion (Chopped)
- About 3.5 tbsp. Cajun Seasoning
- 1 large can of organic diced tomatoes (leave the juice)
- 1 to 2 cloves garlic (Properly Diced)
- About 1 to 2 bay leafs
- About 1 lb. large shrimp, raw & de-veined.
- 2 c. okra (Optional)
- About 4.5 oz. chicken, diced
- 1 package spicy Andouille sausage
- 1/2-1 head of cauliflower
- 5 cups chicken stock.

Directions:

1. First of all, please make sure you have all the ingredients available. Put the chopped peppers, chicken, onions, garlic, Cajun seasoning, Red Hot, & bay leafs in the crockpot with the chicken stock.

2.   Now as you can see, I grabbed a container of my homemade stock directly from the freezer & threw it in.
3.   Set on low for about 6.5 hours.
4.   This step is important. About 30 to 35 minutes before it's finished, toss in the cut up sausages.
5.   Then while this is cooking quickly make cauliflower rice by pulsing raw cauliflower in the food processor until it resembles rice.
6.   Almost there. One thing remains to be done now. For the last 20 to 25 minutes, quickly add in the cauliflower rice & the raw shrimp.
7.   Note: You can choose to quickly steam the cauliflower rice in the microwave & serve the jambalaya over it as well.

Serves: 5 to 6

Time to prepare: 6 hours 30 to 40 minutes (6 hours in crock pot)

Amazing cooking starts here…

Nutritional Information:

Carbohydrates: 12.6g

Protein: 29.2g

Sugar: 5.2g

Saturated Fat: 3.3g

Fat: 16.4g

Calories: 307

Nostalgic Butternut Squash Soup

Don't forget this one…

Ingredients:

- 3 pounds butternut squash, peeled, seeded, and sliced into small chunks
- 1 bay leaf
- 1 cup low-sodium vegetable broth
- About 1 tsp. sea salt
- 1 cup low-sodium chicken broth
- 1 cup sliced shallots
- 3 cloves garlic, minced
- About 2.5 tsp. Extra virgin olive oil
- 1 can (14-ounce) light coconut milk

Optional garnishes:

- Fresh ground black pepper
- Cilantro
- Paprika
- Sunflower seeds

Directions:

1. First of all, please make sure you have all the ingredients available. Preheat your oven to about 440 to 450°F.
2. Now in a rimmed baking sheet, toss together onion, squash, 1 teaspoon oil & salt.

3. Next, quickly roast for about 30 to 35 minutes or until tender & browned.
4. This step is important. Transfer the roasted veggies to a saucepan & add the remaining oil; cook over medium low heat, stirring regularly for about 5 to 10 minutes.
5. Then stir in garlic & cook properly for about 30 to 40 seconds.
6. Almost there. One thing remains to be done now. Stir in coconut milk, broths and bay leaf; cook properly for about 2 to 5 minutes; lower heat & simmer for about 5 to 10 minutes more.
7. Finally discard bay leaf and transfer the mixture to a blender; blend until very smooth. Enjoy.

Servings: 5 to 6

Total Time: 55 to 60 Minutes

Prep Time: 15 to 20 Minutes

Cooking Time: 40 to 45 Minutes

Sizzle your taste buds…

Mighty Quick Mushroom Soup

Legends are born in…

Ingredients:

- About 1 teaspoon sea salt
- 1 large onion (Chopped)
- 2 quarts chicken stock, water or bone broth
- 1 pound shitake mushrooms (Chopped)
- About 2.5 tablespoons olive oil

Directions:

1. First of all, please make sure you have all the ingredients available. Chop onion and mushrooms.
2. Then add oil to a 6-quart pot & heat it over medium heat.
3. Add onion & cook properly for about 15 to 20 minutes, until caramelized.
4. This step is important. Add mushrooms & cook properly for another 5 to 10 minutes, until they become tender.
5. Now add chicken stock & bring to boil. Simmer for about 10 to 15 minutes.
6. Almost there. One thing remains to be done now. Using a hand blender or food processor puree until smooth.
7. Finally serve.

Jaw dropping!!

King sized Baked Chicken And "Rice"

Speed defines it…

Ingredients:

- 1 lb chicken
- About 2.5 tablespoons coconut oil
- 1/3 cup parsley
- 1/4 cup pitted green olives, quartered or halved
- 1 teaspoon paprika
- 3 tablespoons lemon zest
- About 1.5 tablespoon lemon juice
- 3/4 cup chicken stock
- 1 teaspoon onion powder
- 1 teaspoon pepper
- 21/2 teaspoon salt
- 7 cups chopped raw cauliflower
- 1/2 teaspoon garlic powder

Directions:

1. First of all, please make sure you have all the ingredients available. Preheat oven to about 360 to 370 degrees.

2. Now combine cauliflower, parsley, lemon zest, chicken stock, lemon zest, lemon juice, olives, and pepper in a bowl.
3. Spread onto a 9 x 13 inch baking dish that is lined with foil.
4. This step is important. Combine the rest of the seasonings in a bowl & spread all over the available chicken.
5. Then quickly place the chicken pieces on top of the finely chopped cauliflower.
6. Almost there. One thing remains to be done now. Sprinkle any other wanted seasonings on top.
7. Finally bake in the oven for about 40 to 45 minutes, or put in a crockpot and cook properly on low for about 5 to 6 hours.

Mystery with this recipe or rather a chemistry with it.

Crazy Paleo Spicy Beef Curry

Awesomeness fully loaded…

Ingredients:

- 2 Tablespoons curry powder
- About 1 teaspoon sea salt
- 1 medium white onion (Diced)
- About 2.5 Tablespoons chili sauce
- 1/2 inch piece of ginger, peeled and minced
- 2 cups whole fat coconut milk
- 3 garlic cloves (Minced)
- 2.5 pounds beef chuck

Directions:

1. First of all, please make sure you have all the ingredients available. Now place all the ingredients in the crock pot.
2. Almost there. One thing remains to be done now. Then cook properly on low for about 3 to 4 hours.
3. Serve warm. Side with rice, pita bread/naan.

Cooking Time: 3 to 4 hrs

Serving: 8 to 10

Now the wait is over for hungry people.

Nutrition Facts (Per Serving):

8.2g Total Fat

3.5g Saturated Fat

0g Trans Fat

101mg Cholesterol

508m Potassium

2.2g Sugars

237 Calories

4.1g Carbohydrates

385mg Sodium

0.9g Dietary Fiber

34.8g Protein

Pinnacle Raspberry Sorbet

Magical, isn't it?

Ingredients:

- 1/2 medium banana
- 1 egg white
- 1/3 cup coconut milk
- About 1.5 tbsp honey
- About 1.5 tbsp lemon juice
- 1 1/2 cups raspberries

Process:

1. First of all, please make sure you have all the ingredients available. Beat the egg white to stiff peaks.
2. Now put raspberries, honey, banana, coconut milk and lemon juice in a blender, & blend until smooth.
3. Add the mixture gently to the beaten egg white & pour into a freezer proof container.
4. Almost there. One thing remains to be done now. Then freeze for about 6.5 hours or overnight until set.
5. Finally cut into slices before serving.

Cooking time: 10 to 15 minutes + 6 hours to freeze

Servings: 4 to 6 portions

Yeah, it is a vintage recipe.

Perfect Blueberry lemon muffins

Always the upper hand…

Ingredients:

- 1/2 cup coconut oil
- 1 cup fresh blueberries
- About 1.5 tsp pure vanilla extract
- 1/4 tsp baking soda
- 1/4 cup grade B maple syrup
- About 1 tsp salt
- 1 lemon, juice and zest
- 1/2 cup flour
- 6 eggs

Directions:

1. First of all, please make sure you have all the ingredients available. Melt coconut oil in a saucepan.
2. Now mix the eggs, pure vanilla extract, lemon juice, maple syrup, and lemon zest & melted coconut oil.
3. This step is important. Sift in the salt, flour, and baking soda, and blend until smooth.
4. Then add the blueberries. Stir again.
5. Fill 3/4 of the batter into the baking silicon cups.

6. Almost there. One thing remains to be done now. Bake for about 35 to 40 minutes at 340 to 350°F.
7. Finally serve immediately.

It takes: 35 to 40 minutes

You get: 12 to 14 muffins

Now you're happy...?

Dashing Simple Meatballs

Classic style…

Ingredients:

- 1 egg, whisked
- Black pepper to the taste
- 16 ounces canned tomatoes, crushed
- 1 yellow onion (Chopped)
- 14 ounces canned tomato puree
- 2 garlic cloves (Minced)
- 1/4 cup parsley (Chopped)
- 1 and 1/2 pounds beef, ground

Directions:

1. First of all, please make sure you have all the ingredients available. Now in a bowl, mix beef with egg, garlic, parsley, black pepper and onion and stir well.
2. Almost there. One thing remains to be done now. Then shape 16 meatballs, place them in your slow cooker, add tomato puree & crushed tomatoes on top,

cover & cook properly on Low for about 7 to 8 hours.

3.   Finally arrange them on a platter & serve.

Preparation time: 10 to 15 minutes

Cooking time: 8 to 9 hours

Servings: 4 to 6

Arrive in style with this recipe.

Nutritional information:

Fat 5

Carbs 10

Protein 7

Fiber 3

Calories 160

Reliable Fennel Pork Apple Breakfast Patties

Ironic in taste…

Ingredients:

- 2 tsp. Fennel seeds
- 1 tsp. sea salt
- About 3.5 tbsp. coconut oil
- 1/4 tsp. black pepper
- 2 tbsp. Maple syrup
- 450g ground pork (You can use Minced Chicken or Lamb if desired)
- 1/2 tsp. ground sage
- 1 tsp. onion powder
- About 1.5 tsp. garlic powder
- 1/2 tsp. red pepper flakes
- 1 tsp. paprika
- 1/2 tsp. dried rosemary
- 1/2 red apple, diced

Directions:

1. First of all, please make sure you have all the ingredients available. Then toast fennel seeds in a sauté pan set over medium for about 5 to 10 minutes or until fragrant.
2. Almost there. One thing remains to be done now. Now in a large bowl, combine all ingredient except coconut oil; flatten the mixture between your hands to make patties.

3. Finally melt coconut oil in a large skillet set over low heat; add three or four patties & cook properly about 5 to 10 minutes per side or until cooked through and golden brown.

Servings: Eight 2-inch patties

Total Time: 35 to 40 Minutes

Prep Time: 10 to 15 Minutes

Cooking Time: 25 to 30 Minutes

Looking forward to this one!!

Thanks for reading my paleo cookbook.